WHAT'Z SHAKE'N©

I0117117

BRIAN E. STEVENS, Sr.

To order additional copies of this title,
Contact your local bookstore or call 1-888-498-1530 Ext: 101

To purchase in bulk of 10 or more at wholesale prices:
Email: sales.whatzshaken@gmail.com or call: Phone: 1-888-498-1530 Ext: 101

DEDICATION

This book is dedicated to those who are helping people get healthier all around the world, one person at a time. Utilize this book as a resource to increase volume points, add variety to shakes, and increase nutrition club awareness.

CONTENTS

ACKNOWLEDGMENTS

For all those who have been waiting for a one stop shake shop, this resource is for you. Thank you for telling me to hurry up and get it done.

Michelle Dean, Managing Editor, thank you for putting up with my, "Are you done yet?" You simple smile, then say, "I'm so glad you don't believe in micro-management!" You're amazing, beyond words and I appreciate all that you do.

Shaun Morton, thank you for introducing me to the BEST health & wellness company in the WORLD. I'm proud to be an Active World Team member and we're just getting started. "People over Profit" is our motto.

To my family and loved one's. Thank you for believing in me. You taught me in order to achieve greatness, you must first believe you are GREAT! You guys are the ones who are great. I'm just trying to keep up.

Team Herba-Innovators. You're my friends, family members, and business partners. Thank you for allowing me to provide innovative ways to grow as a collective. Even more, I would like to thank each and every one of you for being active business owners. You're getting the world healthier, one person at a time. BRAVO ZULU (good job).

Thank you for allowing me to take empty shake container selfies. I'm pretty sure I'm not the only one who does this, so yes, this is dedicated to all those who place products in the right position, in order to get that perfect photo.

FRENCH VANILLA F1 SHAKES

BANANA BUTTER

2 TBSP. FRENCH VANILLA F1
1-2 TBSP. VANILLA PDM
1 CUP WATER/1 CUP ICE
1 TBSP. BANANA CREAM PUDDING
1 TBSP. PB2 OR NATURAL P BUTTER

HAWIAN DELIGHT

2 TBSP. FRENCH VANILLA F1
1-2 TBSP. VANILLA PDM
1 CUP WATER
1 TBSP. COCONUT SYRUP
1 TBSP. PINEAPPLE JUICE
1 TBSP. ORANGE JUICE

COCO-LOCO

2 TBSP. FRENCH VANILLA F1
1 CUP APPLE JUICE
1 TBSP. COCONUT MILK
1/2 BANANA
1/4 TSP OF GINGER

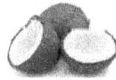

AMERICAN PIE

2 TBSP. FRENCH VANILLA F1
1-2 TBSP. VANILLA PDM
1 CUP APPLE JUICE
1/2 CUP CHOPPED APPLE
1/2 TSP. CINNAMON
DASH NUTMEG

APRICOT

2 TBSP. FRENCH VANILLA F1
1-2 TBSP. VANILLA PDM
1 CUP WATER
6 OZ. APRICOT YOGURT (REDUCED FAT/SUGAR FREE)

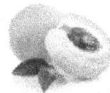

ite BRIAN E. STEVENS SR.

WHITE SANGRIA

2 TBSP. FRENCH VANILLA F1
4 FL. OZ. OF CRYSTAL LIGHT LEMONADE
6 OZ. LIGHT PEACH YOGURT
   (FROZEN, REDUCED SUGAR-FAT FREE) 1/2 OF APRICOT
1/2 OF NECTARINE

ARTIC WILDERNESS

2 TBSP. FRENCH VANILLA F1
1 TBSP. VANILLA PDM
1/2 CUP OF WATER
1/2 PEACH, FROZEN
5 BLUEBERRIES, FROZEN
1/2 TBSP. CRUSHED PECANS
1 TBSP. VANILLA EXTRACT
1/2 CUP LIGHT VANILLA FROZEN YOGURT

BRUISER

2 TBSP. FRENCH VANILLA F1
1/2 CUP APPLE JUICE
1/4 CUP BLUEBERRIES
1/4 CUP BLACKBERRIES
1/2 OF BANANA
1/3 CUP RASPBERRY SHERBET

BANANABERRY TWIST

2 TBSP. FRENCH VANILLA OR WILD BERRY F1
1-2 TBSP. VANILLA PDM
1 CUP WATER 1/2 OF BANANA
1/4 CUP FRESH OR FROZEN BLUEBERRIES/ STRAWBERRIES

RABBIT FOOD

2 TBSP. FRENCH VANILLA F1
1 CUP CARROT JUICE
1/2 CUP APPLE JUICE
6 OZ. NONFAT VANILLA OR PLAIN FROZEN YOGURT
1/2 OF BANANA

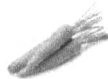

BLUEBERRY

2 TBSP. FRENCH VANILLA F1
1-2 TBSP. VANILLA PDM
1/2 CUP WATER
1/4 CUP BLUEBERRIES (FRESH)
6 OZ. LIGHT PEACH YOGURT

LEMON DROP

2 TBSP. FRENCH VANILLA F1
1-2 TBSP. VANILLA PDM
1 CUP WATER/1 CUP ICE
1 TBSP. LEMON PUDDING MIX

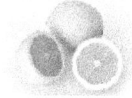

THE CABANNA

2 TBSP. FRENCH VANILLA F1
1/2 OF BANANA
1/2 CUP CRUSHED PINEAPPLE
1/2 CUP NONFAT YOGURT
1 TBSP. HONEY
1 TBSP. COCONUT EXTRACT

FRUIT WAVE

2 TBSP. FRENCH VANILLA F1
1/4 CUP RIPE BANANA
1/4 CUP CHOPPED MANGO
1/4 CUP WHOLE STRAWBERRIES
1/2 CUP PINEAPPLE JUICE
1/2 CUP ORANGE JUICE

FLORIDA SUNBURST

2 TBSP. FRENCH VANILLA F1
1-2 TBSP. VANILLA PDM
3 FL. OZ. FRESH FLORIDA ORANGE JUICE
2 – 5 ICE CUBES
4 OZ. ORANGE LIFT-OFF
·   BLEND FIRST 3 INGREDIENTS
·   ADD ORANGE LIFT-OFF
·   STIR

PINEAPPLE COCO-CRUSH

2 TBSP. FRENCH VANILLA F1
1 -2 TBSP. VANILLA PDM
1/2 CUP WATER
1 – 6 OZ. NONFAT COCONUT YOGURT
1 TBSP. CRUSHED PINEAPPLE
1/2 OF BANANA

GREEN CRUSH

2 TBSP. FRENCH VANILLA F1
1 CUP WATER
1/2 KIWI FRUIT
1/2 BANANA
2 TBSP. CRUSHED PINEAPPLE
2 FL. OZ. MANGO HERBAL ALOE JUICE

ULTIMATE-CITRUS RUSH

2 TBSP. FRENCH VANILLA F1
1/2 CUP DICED PINEAPPLE
1/2 CUP DICED CANTALOUPE
1/2 CUP FRESH ORANGE JUICE
1/2 CUP CARROT JUICE
PINCH OF NUTMEG

ORANGESICLE

2 TBSP. FRENCH VANILLA F1
1-2 TBSP. VANILLA PDM
1 CUP WATER
1 SCOOPS ORANGE H3O

PAPAYA – RASPBERRY

2 TBSP. FRENCH VANILLA F1
1/2 CUP FRUIT JUICE OR WATER
1/2 FROZEN BANANA, PEELED
1/2 CUP FRESH PINEAPPLE
10-12 RASPBERRIES

ITALIAN SODA

2 TBSP. FRENCH VANILLA F1
3 FL. OZ. ORANGE JUICE
3 FL. OZ. SODA WATER
3 FL. OZ. WATER
2 TBSP. HERBAL ALOE JUICE

PEACHSICLE

2 TBSP. FRENCH VANILLA F1
1-2 TBSP. VANILLA PDM
1 CUP WATER
1 PEACH

PEACHES & DREAMS

2 TBSP. FRENCH VANILLA F1
6 FL. OZ. APPLE JUICE
3– 5 SLICES OF PEACH
4 LARGE STRAWBERRIES
1/2 OF BANANA
1/8 TSP CINNAMON

BANANA 'STACHE

2 TBSP. FRENCH VANILLA   F1
1/2 CUP PLAIN NONFAT YOGURT
1 TBSP. PISTACHIO INSTANT PUDDING MIX
1/2 BANANA

PINA COLADA

2 TBSP. FRENCH VANILLA F1
1-2 TBSP. VANILLA PDM
1/2 CUP WATER
1/4 CUP FRESH PINEAPPLE
1 TBSP. COCONUT

PUMPKIN PIE

2 TBSP. FRENCH VANILLA F1
1-2 TBSP. VANILLA PDM
1 CUP WATER
1 TBSP. VANILLA EXTRACT
1/4 TSP. PUMPKIN PIE SPICE

PINEAPPLE BERRY SPLASH

2 TBSP. FRENCH VANILLA F1
1/2 CUP ORANGE JUICE
1/4 CUP PINEAPPLE JUICE
1 PINEAPPLE RING
1/2 CUP MIXED BERRIES
   3 OZ. NONFAT YOGURT (ANY FLAVOR)

SHERBERT JOY

2 TBSP. FRENCH VANILLA OR WILD BERRY F1
6 FL. OZ. WATER
2 SCOOPS SHERBET
   (ORANGE, STRAWBERRY, PINEAPPLE, OR RAINBOW)

VERY BERRY

2 TBSP. FRENCH VANILLA F1
4 FL. OZ. CRYSTAL LIGHT LEMONADE
6 OZ. LIGHT STRAWBERRY YOGURT
(FROZEN, REDUCED SUGAR-FAT FREE)
5 LARGE STRAWBERRIES

STRAWBERRY PARADISE

2 TBSP. FRENCH VANILLA F1
1/2 CUP WHOLE STRAWBERRIES
1 CUP DOLE PINEAPPLE JUICE
1/2 CUP ORANGE JUICE
1/2 CUP LOW FAT VANILLA FROZEN YOGURT

STRAW-ANA

2 TBSP. FRENCH VANILLA F1
1-2 TBSP. VANILLA PDM
1/2 CUP WATER
1/2 CUP APPLE JUICE
4 STRAWBERRIES
1/2 BANANA

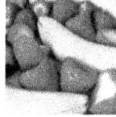

RAY OF SUNSHINE

2 TBSP. FRENCH VANILLA F1
1/2 MEDIUM BANANA
1/2 RIPE PEACH (PEELED, HALVED, PITTED & DICED)
1/2 CUP RASPBERRIES
1/2 CUP ORANGE JUICE

ZESTY SUMMER BLEND

2 TBSP. FRENCH VANILLA F1
1/2 CUP DOLE PINE-ORANGE JUICE
1/2 CUP CRYSTAL LIGHT LEMONADE
1 NECTARINE
6 OZ. LIGHT PEACH YOGURT

EGG NOG

2 TBSP. FRENCH VANILLA F1
2 TBSP. VANILLA PDM
1 C. WATER
1 TBSP. HONEY
1 TBSP. VANILLA EXTRACT
1/8 TSP NUTMEG

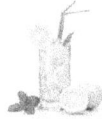

SUMMER TIME

2 TBSP. FRENCH VANILLA F1
1 CUP CRYSTAL LIGHT LEMONADE
1 CUP WATERMELON

KEY LIME PIE

2 TBSP. FRENCH VANILLA F1
1-2 TBSP. VANILLA PDM
1 CUP WATER/1 CUP ICE
1/2 CUP KEY LIME PIE YOGURT
1 TSP LIME JELL-O MIX

ROOT BEER FLOAT

2 TBSP. FRENCH VANILLA F1
1-2 TBSP. VANILLA PDM
1 CUP WATER/1 CUP ICE
1 TBSP. VANILLA PUDDING
1 TBSP. ROOT BEER SYRUP

PRALINES & CREAM

2 TBSP. FRENCH VANILLA F1
1-2 TBSP. VANILLA PDM
1 TSP SUGAR FREE BUTTERSCOTCH PUDDING MIX
1TBSP CHOPPED PECANS
OPTIONAL 1 TSP IMITATION BUTTER

BANANA NUT BREAD

2 TBSP. FRENCH VANILLA   F1
1-2 TBSP. VANILLA PDM
1 CUP WATER/1 CUP ICE
1 TBSP. BANANA CREAM PUDDING
2 TBSP. WALNUTS

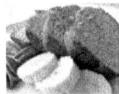

BLUEBERRY MUFFIN

2 TBSP. FRENCH VANILLA   F1
1-2 TBSP. VANILLA PDM
1 CUP WATER/1 CUP ICE
1/2 CUP FROZEN/FRESH BLUEBERRIES
1 TBSP. PISTACHIO SUGAR FREE PUDDING MIX

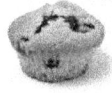

BLUEBERRY LEMON

2 TBSP. FRENCH VANILLA F1
1-2 TBSP. VANILLA PDM
1 CUP WATER/1 CUP ICE
1 TBSP. LEMON SUGAR FREE PUDDING MIX
1/2 CUP FROZEN/ FRESH BLUEBERRIES

WHITE CHOCOLATE RASPBERRY CHEESECAKE

2 TBSP. FRENCH VANILLA F1
1-2 TBSP. VANILLA PDM
2 TBSP. FROZEN RASPBERRY
1 TBSP. WHITE CHOCOLATE SUGAR FREE PUDDING MIX
1 TBSP. CHEESECAKE SUGAR FREE PUDDING MIX

LEMON-BERRY CHEESECAKE

2 TBSP. FRENCH VANILLA F1
1-2 TBSP. VANILLA PDM
1 CUP WATER/1 CUP ICE
1 TBSP LEMON SUGAR FREE PUDDING MIX
1 TBSP. CHEESECAKE SUGAR FREE PUDDING MIX
4 FRESH/FROZEN STRAWBERRIES

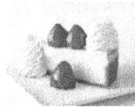

FRENCH TOAST

2 TBSP. FRENCH VANILLA F1
1-2 TBSP. VANILLA PDM
1 C. WATER/1 C. ICE
1 TBSP. VANILLA PUDDING
1 TBSP. MAPLE SYRUP
1 DASH (1/8 TSP.) OF CINNAMON

11

HOPSCOTCH

2 TBSP. FRENCH VANILLA F1
1-2 TBSP. VANILLA PDM
1 CUP WATER/1 CUP. ICE
1 TBSP. BUTTERSCOTCH PUDDING
1 TBSP. CARAMEL SYRUP

STRAWBERRY CHEESECAKE

2 TBSP. FRENCH VANILLA   F1
1-2 TBSP. VANILLA PDM
1 TBSP. SUGAR FREE STRAWBERRY JELL-O
1 TBSP CHEESECAKE SUGAR FREE PUDDING MIX
1/2 GRAHAM CRACKER

CANDY CANE

2 TBSP. FRENCH VANILLA F1
1-2 TBSP. VANILLA PDM
1 CUP WATER
1/2 TBSP. VANILLA PUDDING
1/2 TBSP. PEPPERMINT CHIPS

CHERRY CHEESECAKE

2 TBSP. FRENCH VANILLA F1
1-2 TBSP. VANILLA PDM
1 CUP WATER
1/4 CUP FROZEN CHERRIES
1 TBSP. CHEESECAKE PUDDING MIX

CHERRY COBBLER

2 TBSP. FRENCH VANILLA F1
1-2 TBSP. VANILLA PDM
1 CUP WATER
4 FROZEN CHERRIES
1/4 TSP. CHERRY JELL-O
GRAHAM CRACKER CRUMBS ON TOP

FRENCH VANILLA CAPPUCCINO

2 TBSP. FRENCH VANILLA F1
1-2 TBSP. VANILLA PDM
1 CUP WATER
1 TBSP. VANILLA CAPPUCCINO

LEMON CHEESECAKE

2 TBSP. FRENCH VANILLA F1
1-2 TBSP. VANILLA PDM
1 CUP WATER
1 TBSP. LEMON JUICE
1/2 TBSP. LEMON JELL-O OR LEMONADE CRYSTAL LIGHT
1/2 TBSP. CHEESECAKE PUDDING MIX

ORANGE-ANA

2 TBSP. FRENCH VANILLA F1
8 OZ. ORANGE JUICE (REDUCED SUGAR)
1/2 OF BANANA

PEACH MANGO

2 TBSP. FRENCH VANILLA F1
1-2 TBSP. VANILLA PDM
1 CUP WATER
1-3 FROZEN PEACH SLICES
SMALL HANDFUL OF FROZEN MANGO PIECES
1/2 TBSP. PEACH JELL-O
1 SPLENDA PACKET TO SWEETEN(OPTIONAL)

ROCKY ROAD

2 TBSP. FRENCH VANILLA F1
1-2 TBSP. VANILLA PDM
1 CUP WATER
1 TBSP. CHOCOLATE PUDDING MIX PECANS
MINI MARSHMALLOWS (SUGAR FREE/FAT FREE)

ORANGE JULIUS

2 TBSP. FRENCH VANILLA F1
1-2 TBSP. VANILLA PDM
1 CUP WATER
3 TBSP. FROZEN ORANGE JUICE
1 TBSP. VANILLA EXTRACT
3 ICE CUBES

CRANBERRY CITRUS BLAST

2 TBSP. FRENCH VANILLA F1
1/2 TSP ORANGE EXTRACT
8 FL OZ. ORANGE JUICE
4 TSP HERBAL CRANBERRY ALOE CONCENTRATE
3 ICE CUBES

WILD BERRY F1 SHAKES

SENSATION SHAKE

2 TBSP. WILD BERRY F1
8 FL. OZ. ORANGE JUICE
1/2 OF BANANA

STRAWBERRY DELIGHT

2 TBSP. WILD BERRY F1
1-2 TBSP. VANILLA PDM
1 CUP WATER
1 CUP FROZEN STRAWBERRIES

WILD BERRY ORANGE SUNRISE

2 TBSP. WILD BERRY F1
8 OZ. ORANGE JUICE
1 CUP FROZEN MIXED BERRIES

MANGO BERRY-ANA

2 TBSP. WILD BERRY F1
1-2 TBSP. VANILLA PDM
1 CUP WATER/1 CUP ICE
2 CAPFULS MANGO ALOE CONC.
1 TBSP. VANILLA PUDDING
4 FROZEN STRAWBERRIES
OPTIONAL   1/2 BANANA

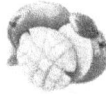

STRAWBERRY FIZZ

2 TBSP. WILD BERRY F1
8 FL. OZ. DIET 7–UP
4 STRAWBERRIES
1/2 OF BANANA

STRAWBERRY BANANA

2 TBSP. WILD BERRY F1
1-2 TBSP. VANILLA PDM
1 CUP WATER/1 CUP ICE
1 TBSP. BANANA CREAM PUDDING
1 TBSP. STRAWBERRY SYRUP
1/4 OF BANANA
2 FROZEN STRAWBERRIES

EXTREME VERY BERRY

2 TBSP. WILD BERRY F1
1-2 TBSP. VANILLA PDM
1 CUP WATER/1 CUP ICE
1/4 CUP MIXED TRIPLE BERRIES
1 TBSP. VANILLA PUDDING

BANANA BERRY

2 TBSP. WILD BERRY F1
1-2 TBSP. VANILLA PDM
1 CUP WATER/1 CUP ICE
1 TBSP. BANANA PUDDING
1/4 CUP TRIPLE BERRIES

BLUEBERRY SENSATION

2 TBSP. WILD BERRY F1
1-2 TBSP. VANILLA PDM
1 CUP WATER/1 CUP ICE
1 TBSP. VANILLA PUDDING
1/4 CUP FROZEN BLUEBERRIES

FRUIT FIZZY

2 TBSP. WILD BERRY F1
4 FL. OZ. UNSWEETENED ORANGE JUICE
1/2 OF BANANA
2 TBSP. STRAWBERRY YOGURT
4 – 6 OZ. DIET 7–UP

MAUI CRUSH

2 TBSP. WILD BERRY F1
2 FL. OZ. HERBAL CRANBERRY ALOE JUICE
2 TBSP. CRUSHED PINEAPPLE
1 TBSP. COCONUT MILK
4 FL. OZ. ORANGE JUICE

BLUEBERRY CHEESECAKE

2 TBSP. WILD BERRY   F1
1-2 TBSP. VANILLA PDM
1 CUP WATER/1 CUP ICE
1 TBSP. CHEESECAKE PUDDING
1/4 CUP BLUEBERRIES

FRUIT BLAST

2 TBSP. WILD BERRY F1
2 – 3 FROZEN STRAWBERRIES
2 - 3 FROZEN PINEAPPLE RINGS
1/4 BANANA
1 CUP ORANGE JUICE

COOKIES AND CREAM F1 SHAKES

NO BAKE COOKIE

1 TBSP. COOKIES & CREAM F1
1 TBSP. DUTCH CHOCOLATE F 1
1-2 TBSP. CHOCOLATE PDM
1 TBSP. PEANUT BUTTER
1 TBSP. QUICK OATS

CINNAMON ROLL

2 TBSP. COOKIES & CREAM F1
1-2 TBSP. VANILLA PDM
1 CUP WATER
1/2 TBSP. BUTTERSCOTCH PUDDING MIX
4 OR 5 DASHES OF CINNAMON
SPLENDA TO TASTE.
1/2 TSP PECANS

OATMEAL CHOCOLATE CHIP COOKIE

2 TBSP. COOKIES & CREAM F1
1-2 TBSP. VANILLA PDM
1 CUP. WATER
1/2 TBSP. VANILLA PUDDING
1/2 TSP. CINNAMON
1 TBSP. QUICK OATS
DASH OF NUTMEG
OPTIONAL 1 TSP. IMITATION BUTTER

WHITE CHOCOLATE REESE'S

2 TBSP. COOKIES & CREAM F1
1-2 TBSP. VANILLA PDM
1 CUP WATER
1 TBSP. OF WHITE CHOCOLATE PUDDING MIX
1 TBSP. OF PEANUT BUTTER PB2

WHAT'Z SHAKE'N

SNAP CRACKLE POP

2 TBSP. COOKIES & CREAM
1-2 TBSP. VANILLA PDM
1 CUP. WATER
3 TBSP. OF RICE KRISPY'S CEREAL
1/2 TBSP. WHITE CHOCOLATE PUDDING
1 TBSP. MARSHMALLOW CREAM
1 SPLENDA PACKET (IF USING REGULAR RICE KRISPY'S)

GIRL SCOUT COOKIE

2 TBSP. COOKIES & CREAM F1
1-2 TBSP. VANILLA PDM
1 CUP WATER
1 TBSP. GRAHAM CRACKER CRUMBS
1 TBSP. COCONUT SHAVINGS
1/2 TBSP. CHOCOLATE FUDGE PUDDING

PEANUT BUTTER PATTIE

2 TBSP. COOKIES & CREAM F1
1-2 TBSP. VANILLA PDM
1 CUP WATER
1 TBSP. GRAHAM CRACKERS
1 TBSP. PEANUT BUTTER
1/2 TBSP. CHOCOLATE FUDGE PUDDING

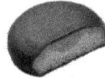

ULTIMATE TURTLE CHEESECAKE

2 TBSP. COOKIES & CREAM F1
1-2 TBSP. VANILLA PDM
1 CUP WATER
1 CAPFUL OF CARAMEL SYRUP (SUGAR FREE/FAT FREE)
1/2 TBSP. CHOC. FUDGE PUDDING
1/2 TBSP. CHEESECAKE PUDDING
1 TBSP. PECANS

SNICKERS

2 TBSP. COOKIES & CREAM F1
1-2 TBSP. VANILLA PDM
1 CUP WATER/1 CUP ICE
1 TBSP. CHOCOLATE SYRUP
1 TSP. VANILLA PUDDING 1 TBSP. PEANUTS
1 TBSP. CARAMEL SYRUP

CHOCOLATE CHIP COOKIE DOUGH

2 TBSP. COOKIES & CREAM F1
1 TBSP. VANILLA PDM
1 TBSP. CHOCOLATE PDM
1 CUP WATER/1 CUP ICE
1/4 CUP CHOCOLATE CHIPS
1 TBSP. PEANUT BUTTER
DASH VANILLA EXTRACT

ICE CREAM SANDWHICH

2 TBSP. COOKIES & CREAM F1
1-2 TBSP. VANILLA PDM
1 CUP WATER/1 CUP ICE
1 TBSP. VANILLA PUDDING
1 TBSP. VANILLA EXTRACT

BANANA SMITH

1 TBSP. COOKIES & CREAM F1
1-2 TBSP. VANILLA PDM
1 CUP WATER/1 CUP ICE
1 TBSP. CHOCOLATE SYRUP
1 TBSP. BANANA PUDDING
4 STRAWBERRIES
1 TBSP. STRAWBERRY JELL-O SUGAR FREE MIX
1/2 BANANA

ALMOND JOY

2 TBSP. COOKIES & CREAM F1
1-2 TBSP. CHOCOLATE PDM
1 CUP WATER
1 TBSP. COCONUT SUGAR FREE PUDDING
1 TBSP. ALMOND EXTRACT

NUTTER BUTTER

2 TBSP. COOKIES & CREAM F1
1-2 TBSP. VANILLA PDM
1 CUP WATER/1 CUP ICE
1 TBSP. PB2
1 TBSP. REAL PEANUT BUTTER
1 TBSP. VANILLA EXTRACT
1/2 TBSP. PEANUT BUTTER SYRUP

BUTTERFINGER

2 TBSP. COOKIES & CREAM F1
1-2 TBSP. CHOCOLATE PDM
1 CUP WATER
1 TBSP. COCONUT SUGAR FREE PUDDING
1 TBSP. ALMOND EXTRACT

SHAUN MORTON SPECIAL

1 TBSP. COOKIES & CREAM F1
1 BANANA CARAMEL F1
10-12 ALMONDS + MINT LEAVES
9 OZ OF WATER
1 TBL. OF ALMOND BUTTER
THEN BLEND

DUTCH CHOCOLATE F1 SHAKES

CAPPUCHINO

2 TBSP. DUTCH CHOCOLATE F1
1-2 TBSP. VANILLA PDM
1/2 CUP WATER
4 OZ. VANILLA FROZEN YOGURT
1 TBSP. INSTANT DECAF COFFEE
DASH CINNAMON

CHOCOLATE BANANA

2 TBSP. DUTCH CHOCOLATE F1
1-2 TBSP. VANILLA PDM
1 CUP WATER
1/2 BANANA

CHOCOLATE ALMOND

2 TBSP. CHOCOLATE F1
1-2 TBSP. VANILLA PDM
1 CUP WATER
1 TBSP. ALMOND EXTRACT

MOCHA CAPPUCHINO

2 TBSP. DUTCH CHOCOLATE F1
1-2 TBSP. VANILLA PDM
1 CUP WATER
1 TBSP. INSTANT CAPPUCCINO

CARAMEL MOCHA CAPPUCHINO

2 TBSP. DUTCH CHOCOLATE F1
1-2 TBSP. VANILLA PDM
1 CUP WATER
1 TBSP. INSTANT CAPPUCCINO MIX
1 TBSP. CARAMEL SYRUP

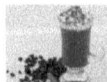

CHOCOLATE COVERED CHERRY

2 TBSP. DUTCH CHOCOLATE F1
1-2 TBSP. VANILLA PDM
1 CUP WATER
1/4 CUP   BLACK CHERRIES

CHOCOLATE MALT

2 TBSP. DUTCH CHOCOLATE F1
1-2 TBSP. VANILLA PDM
1 CUP WATER/1 CUP ICE
1 TBSP. CHOCOLATE SYRUP
1 TBSP. CHOCOLATE PUDDING
1 TBSP. MALT

CHUNKY MONKEY

2 TBSP. DUTCH CHOCOLATE F1
1-2 TBSP. VANILLA PDM
1 CUP WATER
1 TBSP. CHOCOLATE FUDGE PUDDING MIX
1 PROTEIN BAR – PEANUT BUTTER OR CHOC. FUDGE

CHOCOLATE COCONUT DREAM

2 TBSP. DUTCH CHOCOLATE F1
1-2 TBSP. VANILLA PDM
1 CUP WATER
1 TSP OF COCONUT
1/2 TBSP. CHEESECAKE PUDDING MIX
1/2 TBSP. WHITE CHOCOLATE PUDDING MIX

CHOCOLATE RASPBERRY

2 TBSP. DUTCH CHOCOLATE F1
1-2 TBSP. VANILLA PDM
1 CUP WATER
1 CUP FROZEN RASPBERRIES
1 TBSP. ORANGE EXTRACT
4 ICE CUBES

CHOCOLATE COOKIES & CREAM

1 TBSP. DUTCH CHOCOLATE F1
1 TBSP. COOKIES & CREAM F1
1-2 TBSP. VANILLA PDM
1 CUP WATER

CHOCOLATE MINT

2 TBSP. DUTCH CHOCOLATE F1
1-2 TBSP. VANILLA PDM
1 CUP WATER
DASH MINT EXTRACT OR MORE TO TASTE

CHOCOLATE PEANUT BUTTER

2 TBSP. DUTCH CHOCOLATE F1
1-2 TBSP. VANILLA PDM
1 CUP WATER
1 TBSP. CREAMY PEANUT BUTTER

CHOCOLATE PEANUT BUTTER BANANA

2 TBSP. DUTCH CHOCOLATE F1
1-2 TBSP. VANILLA PDM
1 CUP WATER
1 TBSP. CREAMY PEANUT BUTTER
1/2 BANANA

CHOCOLATE COVERED STRAWBERRY

2 TBSP. DUTCH CHOCOLATE
1-2 TBSP. VANILLA PDM
1 CUP WATER
1 CUP FROZEN STRAWBERRIES
1 TBSP. VANILLA EXTRACT
4 ICE CUBES

CRANRASPBERRY DELIGHT

2 TBSP. DUTCH CHOCOLATE F1
1-2 TBSP. VANILLA PDM
8 FL. OZ. CRAN-RASPBERRY JUICE
1/2 OF BANANA

GERMAN CHOCOLATE CAKE

2 TBSP. DUTCH CHOCOLATE F1
1-2 TBSP. VANILLA PDM
1 CUP WATER
1 TBSP. COCONUT SYRUP LIQUEUR
1/2 TBSP. FUDGE PUDDING
1/2 TBSP. PECAN PIECES

MUDSLIDE

2 TBSP. DUTCH CHOCOLATE F1
1-2 TBSP. VANILLA PDM
1 CUP WATER
1/2 TBSP. DAVINCI KAHLUA COFFEE
1 TBSP. INSTANT COFFEE
1 TBSP. SPLENDA

MOCHA ALMOND FUDGE SHAKE

2 TBSP. DUTCH CHOCOLATE F1 1-2 TBSP. VANILLA PDM
1 CUP WATER
1/2 TBSP. CHOCOLATE FUDGE PUDDING
1 TBSP. ALMOND EXTRACT
1 TSP. INSTANT COFFEE
1 SPLENDA PACKET

MOCHA SHAKE

2 TBSP. DUTCH CHOCOLATE F1
1-2 TBSP. VANILLA PDM
1 CUP WATER
1 TSP. INSTANT DECAF COFFEE
1/2 OF BANANA

MOUNDS CHOCOLATE SHAKE

2 TBSP. DUTCH CHOCOLATE F1
1-2 TBSP. VANILLA PDM
1 CUP WATER
1 TBSP. COCONUT EXTRACT
1 TBSP. VANILLA EXTRACT

PEPPERMINT CHOCOLATE

2 TBSP. DUTCH CHOCOLATE F1
1-2 TBSP. VANILLA PDM
1 CUP WATER
2 OZ. VANILLA NONFAT ICE CREAM
1 TBSP. PEPPERMINT EXTRACT

RASPBERRY RAZZMATAZ

2 TBSP. DUTCH CHOCOLATE F1
8 FL. OZ. UNSWEETENED RASPBERRY JUICE
1/3 CUP RASPBERRIES
1/2 OF BANANA

REESE'S CUP

2 TBSP. DUTCH CHOCOLATE F1
1-2 TBSP. VANILLA PDM
1 CUP WATER/1 CUP ICE
1 TBSP. CHOCOLATE   SYRUP
1 TBSP. CHOCOLATE PUDDING
1 TBSP. PEANUTS
1 TBSP. PB2 OR NATURAL PEANUT BUTTER

CAFE LATTE F1 SHAKES

CHOCOLATE CARAMEL LATTE

2 TBSP. CAFÉ LATTE F1
1-2 TBSP. VANILLA PDM
1 CUP WATER/1 CUP ICE
1 TBSP. CHOCOLATE SYRUP
1 TBSP. CHOCOLATE PUDDING
1 TBSP. CARAMEL SYRUP

VANILLA HAZELNUT LATTE

2 TBSP. CAFÉ LATTE F1
1-2 TBSP. VANILLA PDM
1 CUP WATER/1 CUP ICE
1 TBSP. VANILLA PUDDING
1 TBSP. HAZELNUT SYRUP

CHOCOLATE HAZELNUT LATTE

2 TBSP. CAFÉ LATTE F1
1-2 TBSP. VANILLA PDM
1 CUP WATER/1 CUP ICE
1 TBSP. CHOCOLATE SYRUP
1 TBSP. CHOCOLATE PUDDING
1 TBSP. HAZELNUT SYRUP

VANILLA CARAMEL LATTE

2 TBSP. CAFÉ LATTE F1
1-2 TBSP. VANILLA PDM
1 CUP WATER/1 CUP ICE
1 TBSP. VANILLA PUDDING
1 TBSP. CARAMEL SYRUP

MOCHA LATTE

2 TBSP. CAFÉ LATTE F1
1-2 TBSP. VANILLA PDM
1 CUP WATER/1 CUP ICE
1 TBSP. CHOCOLATE SYRUP
1 TBSP. CHOCOLATE PUDDING

PINA COLADA F1 SHAKES

PINA COLADA 2

2 TBSP. PIÑA COLADA F1
1-2 TBSP. VANILLA PDM
1/2 OF BANANA
1 CUP WATER ICE CUBES

CARRIBEAN SUNSET

2 TBSP. PIÑA COLADA F1
1/2 CUP PINEAPPLE SHERBET
1 CUP TROPICAL FRUIT FLAVOR WATER
ICE CUBES

LUAU

2 TBSP. PINA COLADA F1
1 1-2 TBSP. VANILLA PDM
1 CUP WATER
3 FROZEN STRAWBERRIES
1/2 OF BANANA
ICE CUBES

THE DOLI

2 TBSP. PIÑA COLADA F1
1-2 TBSP. VANILLA PDM
1 CUP WATER
2 OZ. PINEAPPLE JUICE
4 FROZEN PINEAPPLE CHUNKS

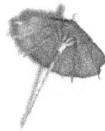

ADDITIONAL FAVORITES

GINGERBREAD COOKIE

2 TBSP. COOKIES AND CREAM F1
1-2 TBSP. VANILLA PDM
1 CUP WATER/1 CUP ICE
1 TBSP. VANILLA PUDDING
1 TBSP. VANILLA SYRUP
1 TBSP. GINGERBREAD SYRUP
1 GINGERBREAD COOKIE (PEPPERIDGE FARM)

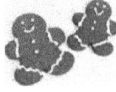

STRAWBERRY MARGARITA

1 TBSP. WILD BERRY F1
1 TBSP. PIÑA COLADA F1
1-2 TBSP. VANILLA PDM
1 CUP WATER/1 CUP ICE
1 TBSP. LEMON PUDDING
1 SCOOP OF LEMONADE H3O
1 TBSP. STRAWBERRY SYRUP
2 STRAWBERRIES
1 TBSP. LIME JUICE

MELON-CHOLY

2 TBSP. TROPICAL FRUIT F1
8 FL OZ. SODA WATER
1/2 CUP FRESH MANGO PIECES
1/2 CUP FRESH CANTALOUPE PIECES
3 ICE CUBES

TURTLE

2 TBSP. DULCE DE LECHE F1
1-2 TBSP. CHOCOLATE PDM
SMALL HANDFUL OF PECANS
1 CUP WATER

ROLO

2 TBSP. DULCE DE LECHE F1
1-2 TBSP. CHOCOLATE PDM
1 CUP WATER

BANANA FOSTER

2 TBSP. DULCE DE LECHE F1
1-2 TBSP. VANILLA PDM
1 TBSP. PEANUT BUTTER
1 TBSP. BANANA SUGAR FREE PUDDING MIX
DASH CINNAMON

CARAMEL APPLE

2 TBSP. DULCE DE LECHE F1
1-2 TBSP. VANILLA PDM
1-2 TBSP. APPLE FIBER
OPTIONAL - DASH CINNAMON

MANGO TANGO

2 TBSP. ORANGE CREAM F1
1-2 TBSP. VANILLA PDM
2-3 CAPFULS MANGO ALOE
OPTIONAL 1-TBSP SUGAR FREE BANANA PUDDING MIX

CAPTAIN CRUNCH

1 TBSP. WILD BERRY F1
1 TBSP. COOKIES & CREAM F1
1-2 TBSP. VANILLA PDM
1 TSP PEANUT BUTTER
3 TBSP. BLUEBERRIES

CRACKER JACK

2 TBSP. DULCE DE LECHE F1
1-2 TBSP. PEANUT BUTTER
OPTIONAL: BUTTERSCOTCH SUGAR FREE PUDDING MIX

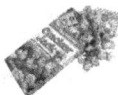

31

MY RECIPES

Create your own recipes and keep track of them here!

_____

_____

_____

_____

_____

_____

_____

_____

_____

_____

_____

_____

_____

_____

_____

_____

MY RECIPES

MY RECIPES

ABOUT THE AUTHOR

Brian Stevens, Sr. is a retired service disability connected veteran, who proudly served a total of 24 years the United States Navy and the United States Army, where he's a proud graduate of the United States Army Officer Candidate School.

Brian has a strong passion for helping others, which lead to the formation of N2B Solutions Group, LLC. a conflict management and leadership assessment firm. (www.n2bsolutionsgroup.com) As Founder and President, Brian continues to change lives and foster peace on a global level, one person at a time.

With strong spiritual faith, Brian decided to join Herbalife© after researching the amazing things the company was doing worldwide. Once presented the marketing plan, off he went with a greater sense of purpose. Promoted to Supervisor in 3 weeks, increasing his team to 60 members within 3 months, and 6 months later, Brian reached Active World Team with 138 team members, 11 Supervisors, members in different countries, and 1 World Team Member (Hello **Amaris.** Job well done. President Team is calling your name).

Brian attributes his business success to focusing on customer service and coaching Team Herba-Innovators to be the best they could be. He always tells his team, "When you place People over Profit, you will be rewarded in more ways than you could ever imagine. Find your warrior, then BEAST IT! Never forget, comfort is the enemy of progression and just as long as you remain active, you're already leading the pact. When you walk towards your goals, your goals are activity walking towards YOU! You ARE what you think you ARE and I see unlimited talent in YOU…. Now, you just have to believe IT in order to achieve IT."